THE PCOS DIET COOKBOOK

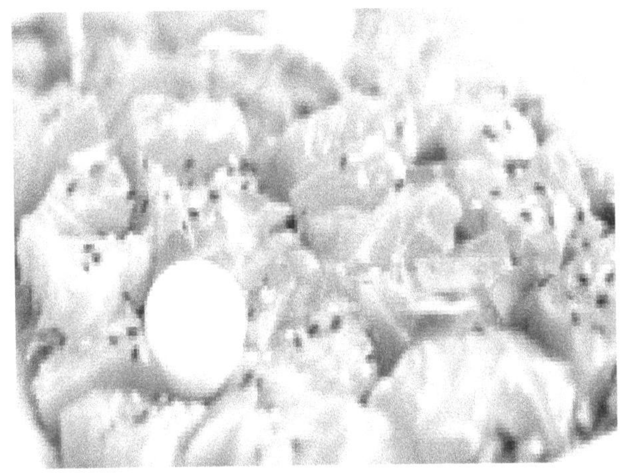

Easy Pcos Recipes For Weight Loss

THERESA EATON

Copyright ©2023 by Theresa Eaton

This book is intended to provide helpful and informative material on the subject matter covered. Every effort has been made to ensure that the information in this book is accurate and up-to-date at the time of the publication. However the author does not warrant that the information contained therein is complete or free from error.

Table of Contents

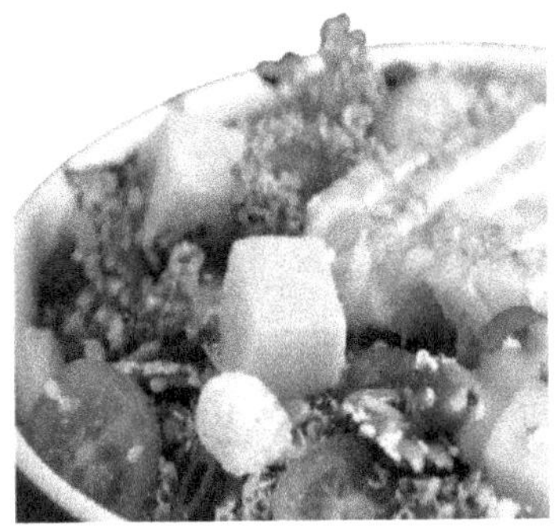

INTRODUCTION

Emily had always had weight issues, but she was never sure why. She had tried every diet under the sun, but nothing had worked. Not until she was given a PCOS diagnosis did anything begin to make sense.

Although Emily was relieved to get an answer at last, she was unsure about her next steps. She decided to try the PCOS Diet Cookbook after hearing about it. She was initially skeptical. She had previously tried a lot of diets, but none of them had been successful. But Emily saw a difference in the PCOS Diet after just a few weeks. She was less bloated than she had previously been and had more energy. She adored the simple recipes and meal preparation advice. She found it easy to follow the diet as a result.

Emily would make the gluten-free banana pancakes for the morning. She ate them all before lunch since they were so filling. She would prepare the quinoa and black bean salad for lunch. It was satisfying and filling.

Emily always struggled to make dinner. Even though she enjoyed cooking, she didn't always have the time or energy to prepare elaborate dinners. With recipes like the turkey meatballs with zucchini noodles from the PCOS Diet Cookbook, it was simple. The recipes were easy to prepare as well as tasty.

Emily adored the wholesome treats and snacks as well. When she had a sweet tooth, she would cook the chocolate chia seed pudding to satisfy her needs without ruining her diet.

Emily has lost 20 pounds after using the PCOS Diet for a few months. She felt more positive and self-assured than she had in a long time. Her alterations to her way of life, such as drinking more water and exercising frequently, had become habits. Emily was appreciative of the PCOS Diet Cookbook's influence on her life. She understood that decreasing weight was important, but so was enhancing her general health. She was eager to follow this direction and see where it would lead her.

CHAPTER 1

Understanding PCOS And Its Impact On Your Health

A hormonal condition known as polycystic ovary syndrome (PCOS) affects millions of women worldwide. It is a syndrome where the ovaries create more male hormones than is typical, which can cause several health problems. Understanding PCOS's implications on your health is crucial because it can affect a woman's physical and mental well-being.

Weight gain or trouble reducing weight is one of the most typical signs of PCOS. Even with diet and exercise, PCOS-afflicted women frequently struggle to lose weight, which can result in other health issues including diabetes and high blood pressure. Acne, excessive hair growth, and hair loss can all be brought on by the ovaries' overproduction of male hormones.

The reproductive health of a woman may be impacted by PCOS. It may be challenging to get pregnant for women with PCOS since they may have erratic or nonexistent menstrual cycles. Ovarian cysts, which can be painful and call for medical attention, are another complication of the illness.

In addition to physical signs, PCOS can have an impact on a woman's psychological state. Depression, anxiety, and mood swings may result from hormonal imbalances linked to PCOS. Due to the physical side effects of the disorder, women with PCOS may also experience problems with their body image and low self-esteem.

Effective PCOS management requires a thorough understanding of the disorder and how it affects your health. Medication, a nutritious diet, and regular exercise can all help manage PCOS symptoms and enhance general health. To manage the emotional effects of the condition, it's also crucial to get help from loved ones and medical specialists.

PCOS is a complicated disorder that may affect a woman's physical and mental health. Effective management of the illness depends on your understanding of how it affects your health. Women with PCOS can have healthy, fulfilling lives with the correct assistance and lifestyle modifications.

The PCOS Diet: What to Eat and What to Avoid

A healthy diet can help manage PCOS symptoms and enhance general health. Blood sugar levels can be balanced, and inflammation in the body can be decreased, with the PCOS diet. To do this, stay away from refined carbohydrates, sugary beverages, and processed foods. Choose entire foods instead, like fresh fruits and vegetables, lean proteins, and healthy fats.

What to eat:

1. Vegetables and fruits: These are a great source of vitamins, minerals, and antioxidants that can assist the body fight inflammation.

2. Lean proteins: To assist regulate blood sugar levels, choose lean proteins such as chicken, turkey, fish, and tofu.

3. Healthy fats: To help lower inflammation and enhance insulin sensitivity, include healthy fats in your diet, such as avocado, nuts, seeds, and olive oil.

4. Whole grains: To help regulate blood sugar levels, choose whole grains such as brown rice, quinoa, and oats rather than processed carbohydrates.

Avoid these foods:

1. Processed foods: These tend to have a lot of sugar, bad fats, and processed carbohydrates, which can make PCOS symptoms worse.

2. Sugary beverages: Steer clear of sugar-filled beverages including soda, juice, and energy drinks that can raise blood sugar levels.

3. Processed carbohydrates: They can lead to blood sugar rises, like white bread, pasta, and pastries.

4. Dairy products: Because some PCOS patients may be sensitive to them, it's recommended to stay away from them or pick low-fat varieties.

Regular exercise is also vital for treating PCOS in addition to a healthy diet. Exercise can help the body become more insulin-sensitive and less inflammatory. Plan to engage in moderate exercise for at least 30 minutes each day, such as brisk walking or cycling.

Women with PCOS can control their symptoms and enhance their general health by avoiding processed meals, sweetened beverages, and refined carbohydrates in favour of nutritious foods like fruits, vegetables, lean proteins, and healthy fats.

Meal Planning and Preparation Tips for PCOS

For women with PCOS, meal planning and preparation can make all the difference. You can make sure you are getting the nutrients your body needs to treat PCOS symptoms and enhance your general health by taking the time to plan and prepare healthy meals.

Here are some suggestions for women with PCOS about food preparation and planning:

1. Schedule your meals ahead of time: Set aside some time each week to schedule your meals for the following week. This will assist you in sticking to your healthy eating objectives and preventing impulsive bad food selections.

2. Opt for whole foods: Pay special attention to whole foods including fruits, vegetables, lean meats, and healthy fats. These meals are nutrient-rich and can aid in managing PCOS symptoms.

3. Make meals in bulk: Making meals in bulk will help you stick to your healthy eating goals while saving time. Prepare wholesome meals in large amounts and freeze them for future use.

4. Use a slow cooker: Making healthy meals quickly and easily is possible with a slow cooker. Just put everything in the morning and let it cook.

5. Keep healthy snacks on hand: When hunger strikes, keep healthy snacks like almonds, seeds, and fresh fruit on hand.

6. Avoid skipping meals: Skipping meals can lead to blood sugar rises and make it more difficult to control PCOS symptoms. Eat frequent, wholesome meals all through the day.

7. Maintain hydration: Drinking plenty of water can assist the body fight inflammation and enhance general health.
Try to drink at least eight glasses of water every single day.

Women with PCOS can take charge of their health and successfully manage their symptoms by adhering to these meal planning and preparation suggestions. Start small and work your way up to a healthy lifestyle, keeping in mind that tiny adjustments can have a major impact on managing PCOS.

CHAPTER 2

BREAKFAST RECIPES

Veggie Omelette

Cooking time: 15 minutes

Servings: 1

Ingredients:

- 2 large eggs
- 1/4 cup chopped vegetables (spinach, bell peppers, mushrooms, etc.)
- 1 tablespoon olive oil
- Salt and pepper to taste

Instructions:

1. In a non-stick skillet, warm up the olive oil over a medium flame.

2. The vegetables should soften after 2–3 minutes of being added and sautéed.

3. Pour the beaten eggs over the sautéed vegetables after seasoning with salt and pepper in a bowl.

4. 3 to 4 minutes should be spent on each side of the omelette to cook until it is set.

5. Serve hot.

Nutritional value (approx.):

Calories: 250 kcal

Protein: 14g

Fat: 18g

Carbohydrates: 5g

Fibre: 2g

Greek Yogurt Parfait

Cooking time: 10 minutes

Servings: 1

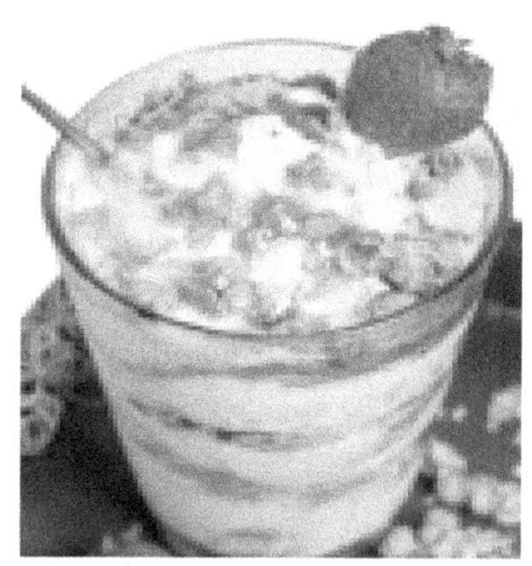

Ingredients:

- 1 cup plain Greek yoghurt
- 1/4 cup fresh berries (strawberries, blueberries, raspberries)
- 1 tablespoon chopped nuts (almonds, walnuts)
- 1 teaspoon honey or stevia (optional)

Instructions:

1. Greek yoghurt, fresh berries, and finely chopped nuts should be arranged in a bowl or glass.

2. Depending on your preference, top with stevia or honey.

3. If you want to repeat the layering.

4. Serve chilled.

Nutritional value (approx.):

Calories: 250 kcal

Protein: 20g

Fat: 10g

Carbohydrates: 20g

Fibre: 4g

Quinoa Breakfast Bowl

Cooking time: 20 minutes

Servings: 2

Ingredients:

- 1/2 cup cooked quinoa
- One cup of non-dairy milk, such as unsweetened almond milk
- 1/2 cup mixed berries
- 2 tablespoons chopped nuts (pistachios, almonds)
- 1 tablespoon chia seeds
- 1 teaspoon honey or stevia (optional)

Instructions:

1. Almond milk and cooked quinoa should be combined in a pot. Cook until thoroughly heated over medium heat.

2. Divide the quinoa mixture into two bowls after taking it off the heat.

3. Add mixed berries, chopped nuts, chia seeds, honey, and/or stevia (if desired) to the top.

4. Serve warm.

Nutritional value (approx.):

Calories: 300 kcal

Protein: 10g

Fat: 15g

Carbohydrates: 35g

Fibre: 8g

Spinach and Mushroom Breakfast Wrap

Cooking time: 15 minutes

Servings: 1

Ingredients:

- 2 large eggs, beaten
- 1 whole wheat tortilla
- 1/4 cup fresh spinach leaves
- 1/4 cup sliced mushrooms
- 1 tablespoon olive oil
- Salt and pepper to taste

Instructions:

1. In a skillet over a medium flame, warm the olive oil.

2. Fry the spinach and mushrooms in the skillet until they are softened and wilted.

3. Vegetables should be taken out of the skillet and put aside.

4. Pour the beaten eggs into the same skillet and scramble them until they are cooked.

5. In a different pan, reheat the whole-wheat tortilla.

Nutritional value (approx.):

Calories: 320 kcal

Protein: 16g

Fat: 18g

Carbohydrates: 25g

Fibre: 4g

Chia Seed Pudding

Cooking time: 5 minutes (plus refrigeration time)

Servings: 2

Ingredients:

- 1/4 cup chia seeds
- One cup of non-dairy milk, such as unsweetened almond milk
- 1 tablespoon honey or stevia
- 1/2 teaspoon vanilla extract
- Fresh berries for topping

Instructions:

1. Chia seeds, almond milk, honey (or stevia), and vanilla extract should all be combined in a bowl. Stir thoroughly.

2. To prevent clumping, give the mixture another stir after 5 minutes.

3. To help the chia seeds absorb the liquid and thicken, cover the bowl and place it in the refrigerator for at least two hours or overnight.

4. When it's time to serve, divide the chia seed pudding among serving bowls and scatter the berries on top.

5. Savour it while chilled.

Nutritional value (approx.):

Calories: 180 kcal

Protein: 5g

Fat: 10g

Carbohydrates: 15g

Fibre: 10g

Sweet Potato Hash

Cooking time: 25 minutes

Servings: 2

Ingredients:

- 1 medium sweet potato, peeled and diced
- 1/2 onion, diced
- 1 bell pepper, diced
- 2 tablespoons olive oil
- 1/2 teaspoon paprika
- Salt and pepper to taste
- 2 eggs (optional)

Instructions:

1. In a skillet over a medium flame, warm up the olive oil.

2. Put the bell pepper, onion, and diced sweet potato in the skillet.

3. Salt, pepper, and paprika should be sprinkled.

4. Cook the sweet potatoes until they are soft and slightly browned, stirring occasionally.

5. Cook the eggs to your liking (optional) in a different pan.

6. If using, place cooked eggs on top of the sweet potato hash before serving.

Nutritional value (approx.):

Calories: 280 kcal

Protein: 5g

Fat: 14g

Carbohydrates: 35g

Fibre: 7g

Berry Smoothie Bowl

Preparation time: 10 minutes

Servings: 1

Ingredients:

- 1 cup frozen mixed berries
- 1/2 ripe banana
- Half a cup of non-dairy milk, such as unsweetened almond milk
- 1 tablespoon almond butter
- Toppings: fresh berries, sliced almonds, shredded coconut, chia seeds

Instructions:

1. Frozen mixed berries, a banana, almond milk, and almond butter should all be combined in a blender.

2. Blend until creamy and smooth.

3. In a bowl, transfer the mixture.

4. Add sliced almonds, shredded coconut, fresh berries, and chia seeds as garnish.

5. Serve right away

Nutritional value (approx.):

Calories: 300 kcal

Protein: 7g

Fat: 15g

Carbohydrates: 35g

Fibre: 10g

Avocado Toast with Poached Eggs

Cooking time: 15 minutes

Servings: 1

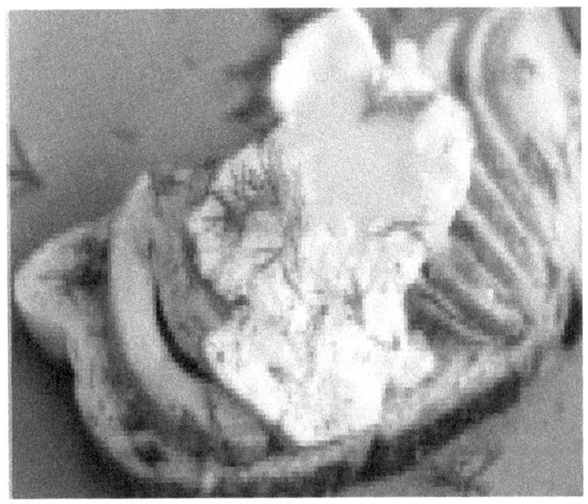

Ingredients:

- 1 slice whole grain bread
- 1/2 ripe avocado, mashed
- 1 poached egg
- Salt and pepper to taste
- Optional toppings: sliced tomatoes, red pepper flakes, chopped herbs

Instructions:

1. Bread should be toasted until golden brown. On the toast, evenly distribute the mashed avocado.

2. Add a poached egg on top.

3. Add salt and pepper to taste.

4. Add any extras you'd like, like diced tomatoes, chilli flakes, or chopped herbs.

5. Serve immediately.

Nutritional value (approx.):

Calories: 320 kcal

Protein: 13g

Fat: 20g

Carbohydrates: 25g

Fibre: 9g

Coconut Flour Pancakes

Cooking time: 20 minutes

Servings: 2-3

Ingredients:

- 1/4 cup coconut flour
- 2 tablespoons almond flour
- 1/2 teaspoon baking powder
- 1/4 teaspoon cinnamon
- Pinch of salt
- 3 large eggs
- A quarter cup of non-dairy milk, like unsweetened almond milk
- 1 tablespoon melted coconut oil
- 1 teaspoon vanilla extract
- Optional toppings: fresh berries, sliced almonds, Greek yoghurt

Instructions:

1. Combine coconut flour, almond flour, baking soda, cinnamon, and salt in a bowl.

2. Beat the eggs in a different bowl. Add vanilla extract, melted coconut oil, and almond milk. Mix thoroughly.

3. After adding the wet ingredients, stir the dry ingredients thoroughly.

4. Allowing the batter to sit will help it thicken.

5. Lightly grease a nonstick skillet or griddle with coconut oil and heat over medium heat.

6. To make pancakes, drop small amounts of batter onto the skillet.

7. Cook until surface bubbles appear, then flip and continue to cook for an additional 1-2 minutes.

8. Continue by using the remaining batter.

9. If desired, top the pancakes with Greek yoghurt, sliced almonds, and fresh fruit.

Nutritional value (approx.):

Calories: 220 kcal (per serving, 3 servings total)

Protein: 9g

Fat: 14g

Carbohydrates: 13g

Fibre: 6g

Almond Flour Blueberry Muffins

Cooking time: 25 minutes

Servings: 6 muffins

Ingredients:

- 1 cup almond flour
- 1/4 cup coconut flour
- 1/4 teaspoon baking soda
- 1/4 teaspoon salt
- 2 tablespoons coconut oil, melted
- 3 tablespoons honey or maple syrup
- 2 large eggs
- 1/2 teaspoon vanilla extract
- 1/2 cup fresh or frozen blueberries

Instructions:

1. Set the oven's temperature to 350°F (175°C). Organize a muffin pan with paper liners.

2. Almond flour, coconut flour, baking soda, and salt should all be combined in a bowl.

3. Melted coconut oil, honey, maple syrup, eggs, and vanilla extract should all be combined in a different bowl. Mix thoroughly.

4. Just combine the dry ingredients with the addition of the wet ingredients.

5. Fold the blueberries in slowly. To fill the muffin tins evenly, divide the batter.

6. 18 to 20 minutes of baking time should yield a muffin with a toothpick inserted in the centre that comes out clean.

7. The muffins should cool in the pan for a few minutes before being moved to a wire rack to finish cooling.

8. As a delicious and filling breakfast option, serve the muffins.

Nutritional value (approx.):

Calories: 220 kcal (per muffin)

Protein: 7g

Fat: 16g

Carbohydrates: 14g

Fibre: 4g

CHAPTER 3

Grilled Chicken Breast with Roasted Vegetables

Cooking Time: 40 minutes

Servings: 2

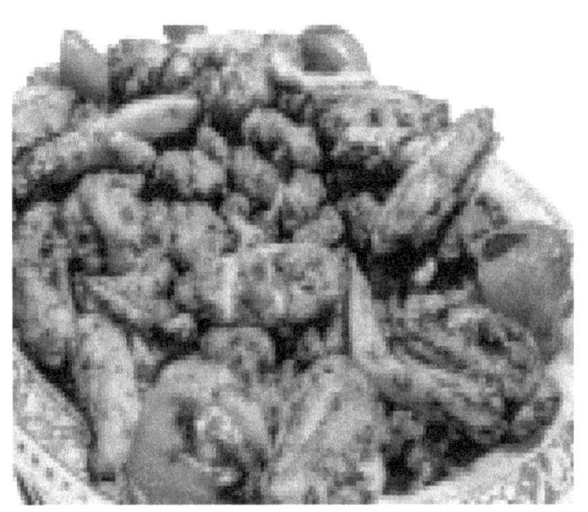

Ingredients:

- 2 boneless, skinless chicken breasts
- 1 medium zucchini, sliced
- 1 medium bell pepper, sliced
- 1 small red onion, sliced
- 2 tablespoons olive oil
- One teaspoon of dried herbs, like thyme, oregano, or rosemary
- Salt and pepper to taste

Instructions:

1. Set the oven's temperature to 400°F (200°C).

2. Salt, pepper, and dried herbs should be used to season the chicken breasts.

3. The chicken breasts should be cooked through after being grilled for 4-5 minutes on each side in a hot grill pan.

4. In the meantime, arrange the red onion, bell pepper, and zucchini slices on a baking sheet.

5. Sprinkle with salt, pepper, and olive oil before tossing to coat.

6. Vegetables should be roasted in a preheated oven for 15 to
    20 minutes, or until they are tender.

7. Serve the roasted vegetables alongside the grilled chicken
    breast.

Approximate Nutritional Value per Serving:

Calories: 320

Protein: 30g

Carbohydrates: 10g

Fat: 18g

Fibre: 4g

Chickpea Salad

Cooking Time: 15 minutes

Servings: 2

Ingredients:

- 1 can chickpeas, drained and rinsed
- 1/2 cup cucumber, diced
- 1/2 cup cherry tomatoes, halved
- 1/4 cup red onion, diced
- 1/4 cup fresh parsley, chopped
- 2 tablespoons lemon juice
- 2 tablespoons extra-virgin olive oil
- Salt and pepper to taste

Instructions:

1. The chickpeas, cucumber, cherry tomatoes, red onion, and parsley should all be combined in a big bowl.

2. In a little container, combine the lemon juice, olive oil, salt, and pepper.

3. After adding the dressing, gently toss the chickpea salad to combine.

4. Enjoy the salad after dividing it into two portions.

Approximate Nutritional Value per Serving:

Calories: 250

Protein: 10g

Carbohydrates: 30g

Fat: 10g

Fibre: 9g

Sweet Potato and Spinach Frittata

Cooking Time: 40 minutes

Servings: 4

Ingredients:

- 4 large eggs

- 1 medium sweet potato, peeled and diced

- 2 cups fresh spinach leaves

- 1/2 cup diced red bell pepper

- 1/4 cup diced onion

- 2 tablespoons olive oil

- 1/4 teaspoon garlic powder

- Salt and pepper to taste

Instructions:

1. Set the oven's temperature to 375°F (190°C).

2. In a skillet that can be used in the oven, warm up the olive oil. Include the sweet potato, onion and bell pepper. For about 8 to 10 minutes, sauté until the sweet potato is tender.

3. To the skillet, add the spinach leaves, and stir frequently till wilted.

4. Eggs, garlic powder, salt, and pepper should all be combined in a bowl.

5. Over the vegetables in the skillet, pour the egg mixture.

6. Bake the frittata for 15-20 minutes, or until it is set and lightly golden, in the preheated oven.

7. Serve the frittata by cutting it into wedges.

Approximate Nutritional Value per Serving:

Calories: 220

Protein: 10g

Carbohydrates: 18g

Fat: 12g

Fibre: 4g

Salmon Salad with Avocado Dressing

Cooking Time: 20 minutes

Servings: 2

Ingredients:

- 2 salmon fillets
- 4 cups mixed salad greens
- 1/2 cucumber, sliced

- 1/4 cup cherry tomatoes, halved

- 1/4 cup red onion, thinly sliced

- 1 ripe avocado

- 2 tablespoons lime juice

- 2 tablespoons Greek yoghurt

- 1 tablespoon extra-virgin olive oil

- Salt and pepper to taste

Instructions:

1. Set the oven's temperature to 400°F (200°C).

2. Add salt and pepper to the salmon fillets. They should be baked for 12 to 15 minutes, or until fully cooked, on a baking sheet.

3. Combine the avocado, lime juice, Greek yoghurt, olive oil, salt, and pepper in a blender or food processor. The avocado dressing is prepared by blending all ingredients until completely smooth.

4. Combine the cooked salmon, mixed salad greens, cucumber, cherry tomatoes, and red onion in a big bowl.

5. Over the salad, drizzle the avocado dressing and give it a gentle toss to combine.

6. Enjoy the salad after dividing it into two portions.

Approximate Nutritional Value per Serving:

Calories: 350

Protein: 25g

Carbohydrates: 15g

Fat: 23g

Fibre: 8g

Turkey and Vegetable Stir-Fry

Cooking Time: 25 minutes

Servings: 2

Ingredients:

- 8 ounces lean ground turkey
- Two cups of a variety of vegetables, such as carrots, broccoli, and bell peppers
- 2 cloves garlic, minced
- 2 tablespoons low-sodium soy sauce
- 1 tablespoon sesame oil
- 1 tablespoon fresh ginger, grated
- 1/4 teaspoon red pepper flakes (optional)
- Salt and pepper to taste

Instructions:

1. Sesame oil should be heated in a sizable skillet or wok over medium heat. Add the ground turkey and cook it until it is browned.

2. Garlic, ginger, soy sauce, red pepper flakes (if using), salt, and pepper should all be added to the skillet along with the mixed vegetables. Stir-fry the vegetables for 5 to 7 minutes, or until they are crisp-tender.

3. If necessary, adjust the seasoning.

4. Serve the stir-fry hot after dividing it into two portions.

Approximate Nutritional Value per Serving:

Calories: 280

Protein: 24g

Carbohydrates: 16g

Fat: 13g

Fibre: 6g

Greek Salad with Grilled Shrimp

Cooking Time: 20 minutes

Servings: 2

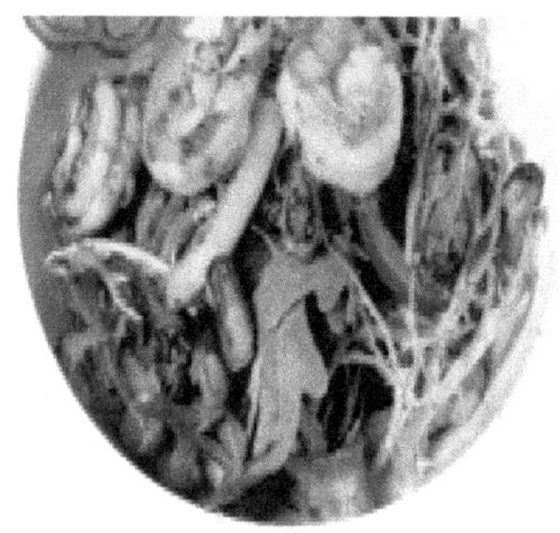

Ingredients:

- 8 ounces shrimp, peeled and deveined
- 4 cups mixed salad greens
- 1/2 cup cherry tomatoes, halved
- 1/4 cup cucumber, sliced
- 1/4 cup red onion, thinly sliced
- 1/4 cup Kalamata olives
- 2 tablespoons crumbled feta cheese
- 2 tablespoons lemon juice
- 2 tablespoons extra-virgin olive oil
- 1 teaspoon dried oregano
- Salt and pepper to taste

Instructions:

1. The grill or grill pan should be heated to a medium-high temperature.

2. Add dried oregano, salt, and pepper to the shrimp before serving. The shrimp should be cooked through after 2 to 3 minutes on each side of the grill.

3. Salad greens, cherry tomatoes, cucumber, red onion, Kalamata olives, and crumbled feta cheese should all be combined in a big bowl.

4. In a small container, mix the salt, pepper, lemon juice, and olive oil.

5. Over the salad, drizzle the dressing, and toss just enough to combine.

6. Grilled shrimp should be placed on top of each of the two portions of the salad.

Approximate Nutritional Value per Serving:

Calories: 290

Protein: 25g

Carbohydrates: 12g

Fat: 16g

Fibre: 4g

Spinach and Mushroom Quiche

Cooking Time:45 minutes

Servings:4

Ingredients:

- 1 ready-made pie crust
- 4 large eggs
- 1 cup fresh spinach, chopped
- 1 cup mushrooms, sliced
- 1/2 cup shredded mozzarella cheese
- 1/4 cup diced onion
- 1/4 cup milk (any type you prefer)
- 1 tablespoon olive oil
- Salt and pepper to taste

Instructions:

1. Set the oven's temperature to 375°F (190°C).

2. Set aside the pie crust n a pie plate.

3. A skillet with olive oil in it should be heated to a medium temperature.

4. Add the mushrooms and onions, and cook them until they are soft and all liquid has been absorbed.

5. In a mixing container, combine the milk and eggs and whisk.

6. Add salt and pepper to taste.

7. Over the entire bottom of the pie crust, distribute the chopped spinach evenly.

8. Add the fried onions and mushrooms on top.

9. Over the vegetables in the pie crust, pour the egg mixture.

10. Shredded mozzarella cheese should be added.

11. Bake the quiche in the preheated oven for 30-35 minutes, or until it is set and the top is lightly golden.

12. Before slicing and serving, take it out of the oven and let it cool for a while.

Approximate Nutritional Value per Serving:

Calories: 320

Protein: 14g

Carbohydrates: 23g

Fat: 19g

Fibre: 2g

Mediterranean Wrap

Cooking Time: 15 minutes

Servings: 2

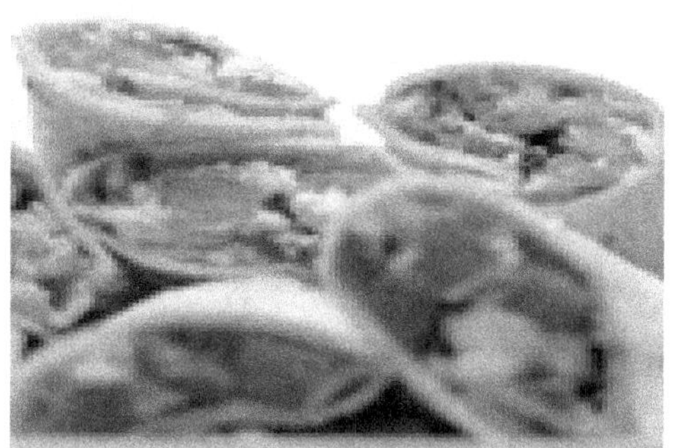

Ingredients:

- 2 whole wheat tortillas or wraps
- 1 cup cooked chicken breast, sliced
- 1/2 cup chopped cucumber
- 1/2 cup diced tomatoes
- 1/4 cup sliced black olives
- 1/4 cup crumbled feta cheese
- 2 tablespoons hummus
- 2 tablespoons plain Greek yoghurt
- Fresh parsley, chopped (for garnish)
- Salt and pepper to taste

Instructions:

1. Lay the tortillas or wrap them flat on a fresh surface as directed.

2. Each tortilla should have an even layer of hummus on it, with a thin border all the way around.

3. Over the hummus, arrange the thinly sliced chicken breast, cucumber, tomatoes, black olives, and crumbled feta cheese.

4. Over the fillings, drizzle plain Greek yoghurt.

5. To taste, add salt and pepper to the food.

6. To add flavour and garnish, top the fillings with fresh parsley.

7. The tortillas' sides should be folded inward before being tightly rolled into wraps.

8. Serve the wraps by cutting them in half.

Approximate Nutritional Value per Serving:

Calories: 350

Protein: 27g

Carbohydrates: 29g

Fat: 14g

Fibre: 5g

Spicy Shrimp Stir-Fry

Cooking Time: 20 minutes

Servings: 2

Ingredients:

- 8 ounces shrimp, peeled and deveined
- Two cups of mixed vegetable varieties such as broccoli, bell peppers, and snap peas
- 1 tablespoon olive oil
- 2 cloves garlic, minced
- 1 teaspoon ginger, grated
- 2 tablespoons low-sodium soy sauce
- One teaspoon of Sriracha sauce, (adjust to your taste for spice)
- Salt and pepper to taste

Instructions:

1. In a sizable skillet or wok, heat the olive oil over a medium-high temperature.

2. To the skillet, add the minced garlic and the grated ginger, and cook until fragrant, about a minute.

3. Cook the shrimp in the skillet for three to four minutes, or until they are opaque and pink.

4. The mixed vegetables should be tender-crisp after 3–4 minutes of cooking after being stirred in.

5. Combine soy sauce and Sriracha sauce in a small bowl.

6. After thoroughly coating the shrimp and vegetables, pour the sauce over them.

7. To taste, add salt and pepper to the food. Cook for one to two more minutes.

8. Serve hot after removing from heat.

Nutritional Value (per serving):

Calories: 250 kcal

Protein: 30g

Fat: 9g

Carbohydrates: 15g

Fibre: 5g

Quinoa Salad with Avocado and Chicken

Cooking Time: 30 minutes

Servings: 2

Ingredients:

- 1 cup cooked quinoa
- 1 cup cooked chicken breast, diced
- 1 avocado, peeled and diced
- 1/2 cup cherry tomatoes, halved
- 1/4 cup red onion, finely chopped
- 1/4 cup fresh cilantro, chopped
- 2 tablespoons lemon juice
- 1 tablespoon olive oil
- Salt and pepper to taste

Instructions:

1. Cooked quinoa, diced chicken breast, avocado, cherry tomatoes, red onion, and cilantro should all be combined in a big bowl.

2. In a different small bowl, mix the salt, pepper, lemon juice and olive oil.

3. Toss the quinoa salad gently after adding the dressing.

4. Serve the salad right away after dividing it into two portions.

Nutritional Value per Serving:

Calories: 400

Protein: 30g

Carbohydrates: 30g

Fat: 20g

Fibre: 10g

CHAPTER 4

SATISFYING DINNER RECIPES

Spicy Turkey Lettuce Wraps

Cooking Time: 25 minutes

Servings: 4

Ingredients:

- 1 pound ground turkey
- 2 tablespoons low-sodium soy sauce
- 1 tablespoon sesame oil
- 1 tablespoon sriracha sauce
- 1 teaspoon minced ginger
- 2 cloves garlic, minced
- 1 cup shredded carrots
- 1/4 cup chopped green onions
- 8 large lettuce leaves

Instructions:

1. The ground turkey should be cooked in a skillet over a medium flame until browned.

2. Mix the soy sauce, sesame oil, sriracha sauce, minced ginger, and minced garlic in a small bowl.

3. Stir well after adding the sauce mixture to the skillet's cooked turkey.

4. To the skillet, add the green onions and carrots that have been chopped.

5. Vegetables should be cooked for 3–4 minutes until they are tender.

6. Fill lettuce leaves with the turkey mixture, then roll them up like a wrap.

7. Serve right away.

Nutritional Value per Serving:

Calories: 210

Protein: 23g

Carbohydrates: 7g

Fat: 10g

Chicken Stir-Fry with Vegetables

Cooking Time: 25 minutes

Servings: 3

Ingredients:

- 2 chicken breasts, sliced
- 2 tablespoons soy sauce (low-sodium)
- 2 tablespoons oyster sauce
- 1 tablespoon sesame oil
- 1 tablespoon cornstarch
- 1 tablespoon olive oil
- 1 red bell pepper, sliced
- 1 yellow bell pepper, sliced
- 1 cup broccoli florets
- 1 cup snap peas
- 2 cloves garlic, minced
- 1 teaspoon grated ginger
- Salt and pepper to taste

Instructions:

1. Combine the soy sauce, oyster sauce, sesame oil, cornstarch, salt, and pepper in a small bowl. Place aside.

2. In a sizable skillet or wok, heat the olive oil over medium-high heat.

3. Sliced chicken breast should be added to the skillet and cooked through. Remove from the skillet and place on one side.

4. Add grated ginger and minced garlic to the same skillet. Sauté until fragrant for one minute.

5. Broccoli florets, snap peas, and bell pepper slices should all be added to the skillet.

6. Vegetables should be cooked for 3–4 minutes to reach crisp–tenderness.

7. Place the cooked chicken back in the skillet with the vegetables, then top with the sauce mixture. To evenly coat everything, thoroughly stir.

8. Cook the ingredients for a further 2 to 3 minutes, or until the sauce thickens and covers everything.

9. Pour over cooked brown rice or cauliflower rice, and serve hot.

Nutritional Value per Serving:

Calories: 320

Protein: 28g

Carbohydrates: 20g

Fat: 12g

Lentil and Vegetable Curry

Cooking Time: 40 minutes

Servings: 4

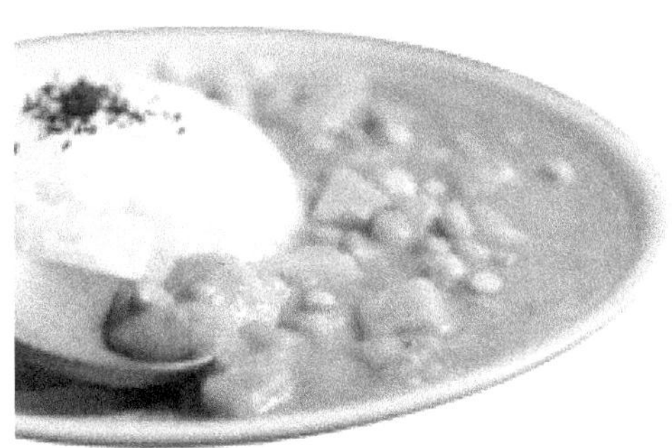

Ingredients:

- 1 cup dried lentils, rinsed
- 1 tablespoon olive oil
- 1 onion, chopped
- 2 cloves garlic, minced
- 1 teaspoon grated ginger
- 1 tablespoon curry powder
- 1 teaspoon ground cumin
- 1 teaspoon ground turmeric
- 1 can diced tomatoes
- 1 cup vegetable broth
- 1 cup chopped spinach
- Salt and pepper to taste
- Fresh cilantro for garnish (optional)

Instructions:

1. The lentils should be cooked as directed on the package until tender. Place aside.

2. The olive oil should be warmed up in a sizable skillet over medium heat.

3. To the skillet, add the minced garlic, grated ginger, and the chopped onion.

4. The onion should be translucent after 3 to 4 minutes of sautéing.

5. Stir in the turmeric, cumin, and curry powder in the skillet.

6. The spices should be thoroughly mixed into the onion mixture.

7. Add the vegetable broth and diced tomatoes. Stir, to mix.

8. To allow the flavours to meld, add cooked lentils to the skillet and simmer for 15 to 20 minutes.

9. Add the spinach, stir, and cook for an additional two to three minutes, or until wilted.

10. To taste, add salt and pepper to the food.

11. If desired, garnish with fresh cilantro.

12. Serve alongside quinoa or brown rice.

Nutritional Value per Serving:

Calories: 290

Protein: 16g

Carbohydrates: 45g

Fat: 5g

Zucchini Noodles Shrimp Scampi

Cooking Time: 20 minutes

Servings: 2

Ingredients:

- 2 medium zucchinis, spiralized into noodles
- 8 ounces shrimp, peeled and deveined
- 2 tablespoons olive oil
- 4 cloves garlic, minced
- 1 tablespoon lemon juice
- 1/4 cup low-sodium chicken broth
- Salt and pepper to taste
- Chopped parsley for garnish (optional)

Instructions:

1. The olive oil should be warmed up in a sizable skillet over medium heat.

2. Add the finely chopped garlic to the skillet and cook for one to two minutes after it becomes fragrant.

3. Cook the shrimp in the skillet for two to three minutes, or until pink and fully cooked.

4. The shrimp should be taken out of the skillet and put aside.

5. Add zucchini noodles to the same skillet and cook for 2–3 minutes, or until tender.

6. The skillet should now contain the cooked shrimp. Add chicken broth and lemon juice. To combine, thoroughly stir.

7. To fully reheat, cook for an additional 2 to 3 minutes.

8. To taste, add salt and pepper to the food. If desired, add chopped parsley as a garnish.

9. Distribute the shrimp scampi with zucchini noodles among serving bowls.

10. Serve right away as a flavorful and light dinner option.

Nutritional Value per Serving:

Calories: 230

Protein: 20g

Carbohydrates: 10g

Fat: 12g

Baked Chicken and Vegetable Foil Packets

Cooking Time: 30 minutes

Servings: 4

Ingredients:

- 4 boneless, skinless chicken breasts
- 2 tablespoons olive oil
- 2 cloves garlic, minced
- 1 teaspoon dried basil
- 1 teaspoon dried oregano
- Salt and pepper to taste
- 1 zucchini, sliced
- 1 yellow squash, sliced
- 1 red bell pepper, sliced

- 1 cup cherry tomatoes, halved

- Fresh parsley for garnish (optional)

Instructions:

1. Set the oven's temperature to 400°F (200°C).

2. Make four sizable aluminium foil pieces. Each chicken breast should be placed on its piece of foil.

3. Olive oil, minced garlic, dried basil, dried oregano, salt, and pepper should all be combined in a small bowl.

4. The olive oil mixture should be brushed on the chicken breasts, coating both sides.

5. Around the chicken, distribute the sliced zucchini, yellow squash, red bell pepper, and cherry tomatoes among the foil packets.

6. To create packets, fold the foil over the chicken and vegetables and seal it tightly.

7. When the chicken is cooked through and the vegetables are tender, place the foil packets on a baking sheet and bake in the preheated oven for 25 to 30 minutes.

8. Open the foil packets carefully, if desired, garnish with fresh parsley, and then serve.

Nutritional Value per Serving:

Calories: 280

Protein: 32g

Carbohydrates: 9g

Fat: 12g

Cauliflower Fried Rice with Tofu

Cooking Time: 25 minutes

Servings: 4

Ingredients:

- 1 small head of cauliflower, grated into a rice-like texture
- 8 ounces firm tofu, drained and diced
- 2 tablespoons sesame oil
- 2 cloves garlic, minced
- One cup of mixed vegetables including corn, peas and carrots.
- 2 tablespoons low-sodium soy sauce

- 1 tablespoon rice vinegar

- 2 green onions, sliced

- Salt and pepper to taste

Instructions:

1. In a sizable skillet or wok, warm the sesame oil over medium heat.

2. Add the finely chopped garlic to the skillet and cook for one to two minutes after it becomes fragrant.

3. Cook the diced tofu in the skillet for 5–6 minutes, or until it begins to lightly brown.

4. When the mixed vegetables are tender, add them to the skillet and cook for an additional 3–4 minutes.

5. To make room for the cauliflower rice, push the tofu and vegetable mixture to one side of the skillet.

6. Cauliflower should be cooked and tender after 3–4 minutes, so add it to the empty side of the skillet and cook it that way.

7. In a little bowl, mix the soy sauce and rice vinegar. Stir everything together thoroughly before adding the mixture to the skillet.

8. To fully reheat, cook for an additional 2 to 3 minutes.

9. To taste, add salt and pepper to the food.

10. As a healthy substitution for conventional fried rice, garnish with thinly sliced green onions and serve.

Nutritional Value per Serving:

Calories: 200

Protein: 13g

Carbohydrates: 12g

Fat: 12g

Baked Cod with Roasted Vegetables

Cooking Time: 30 minutes

Servings: 2

Ingredients:

- 2 cod fillets
- 2 tablespoons lemon juice
- 1 tablespoon olive oil

- 1 teaspoon dried dill

- Salt and pepper to taste

- 1 cup broccoli florets

- 1 cup cauliflower florets

- 1 cup cherry tomatoes

- 1 tablespoon balsamic vinegar

Instructions:

1. Set the oven's temperature to 400°F (200°C).

2. Cod fillets should be placed in a baking dish with lemon juice and olive oil drizzled over them.

3. Over the cod fillets, season with salt, pepper, and dried dill.

4. Place the broccoli florets, cauliflower florets, and cherry tomatoes on a different baking sheet.

5. Olive oil and balsamic vinegar should be poured over the dish after adding salt and pepper.

6. Put the vegetable baking sheet and the baking dish with the cod fillets in the oven.

7. Bake the cod and vegetables for 20 minutes, or until they are both cooked through.

8. Serve the roasted vegetables alongside the baked cod.

Nutritional Value per Serving:

Calories: 230

Protein: 30g

Carbohydrates: 11g

Fat: 8g

Thai Chicken Salad

Cooking Time: 20 minutes

Servings: 2

Ingredients:

- 2 chicken breasts, grilled and sliced
- 4 cups mixed salad greens
- 1 cup shredded cabbage
- 1 carrot, julienned
- 1/2 cucumber, sliced
- 1/4 cup chopped fresh cilantro
- 1/4 cup chopped fresh mint
- 2 tablespoons lime juice
- 1 tablespoon low-sodium soy sauce

- 1 tablespoon honey

- 1 tablespoon peanut butter

- 1 teaspoon grated ginger

- 1 clove garlic, minced

- Salt and pepper to taste

- Crushed peanuts for garnish (optional)

Instructions:

1. Mix salad greens, shredded cabbage, carrot, cucumber, cilantro, and mint in a sizable bowl.

2. To make the dressing, combine the lime juice, soy sauce, honey, peanut butter, minced garlic, ginger, and salt and pepper in a separate small bowl.

3. Sliced grilled chicken should be included in the salad mixture.

4. To evenly coat the salad, drizzle the dressing over it and toss to combine.

5. Crushed peanuts can be used as a garnish if preferred.

6. For a light and filling meal, serve Thai chicken salad.

Nutritional Value per Serving:

Calories: 280

Protein: 30g

Carbohydrates: 21g

Fat: 9g

Baked Lemon Herb Chicken Thighs

Cooking Time: 35 minutes

Servings: 4

Ingredients:

- 4 bone-in, skin-on chicken thighs
- 2 tablespoons lemon juice
- 1 tablespoon olive oil
- 2 cloves garlic, minced
- 1 teaspoon dried thyme
- 1 teaspoon dried rosemary
- Salt and pepper to taste

Instructions:

1. Set the oven's temperature to 400°F (200°C).

2. Mix the lemon juice, olive oil, minced garlic, dried thyme, dried rosemary, salt, and pepper in a small bowl.

3. On a parchment paper-lined baking sheet, put the chicken thighs.

4. The chicken thighs should be covered with the lemon-herb mixture.

5. Cook the chicken in the preheated oven for 30-35 minutes, or until the skin is crispy and the meat is thoroughly cooked.

6. Serve alongside steamed veggies or a side salad

Nutritional Value per Serving:

Calories: 280

Protein: 24g

Carbohydrates: 2g

Fat: 20g

Turkey Meatballs with Zucchini Noodles

Cooking Time: 40 minutes

Servings: 4

Ingredients:

- 1 pound lean ground turkey
- 1/4 cup almond flour

- 1/4 cup grated Parmesan cheese

- 1/4 cup chopped fresh parsley

- 1 egg

- 2 cloves garlic, minced

- 1 teaspoon dried oregano

- Salt and pepper to taste

- 4 medium zucchinis, spiralized into noodles

- 2 cups marinara sauce

Instructions:

1. Set the oven's temperature to 375°F (190°C).

2. Ground turkey, almond flour, grated Parmesan cheese, parsley, egg, minced garlic, dried oregano, salt, and pepper should all be combined in a big bowl.

3. Combine ingredients thoroughly until they are distributed evenly.

4. Make meatballs out of the turkey mixture that is about an inch in diameter.

5. Place the balls of meat in a single layer on a baking sheet that has been lined with parchment.

6. Cook the meatballs in the preheated oven for 20 to 25 minutes, or until they are thoroughly heated through.

7. Heat the marinara sauce in a saucepan over medium heat while the meatballs bake.

8. When the meatballs are finished cooking, add them to the sauce-filled pan and simmer for 5 to 10 minutes to let the flavours meld.

9. Heat a small amount of olive oil over medium heat in a different, big skillet.

10. Spiralized zucchini noodles should be added to the skillet and cooked for 3 to 4 minutes, or until tender.

11. Along with zucchini noodles and marinara sauce, serve the turkey meatballs.

Nutritional Value per Serving:

Calories: 270

Protein: 26g

Carbohydrates: 14g

Fat: 12g

CHAPTER 5

HEALTHY SNACKS AND DESSERTS

Yogurt Parfait

Preparation time: 5 minutes

Servings: 1

Ingredients:

- 1 cup plain Greek yoghurt
- 1/4 cup mixed berries (such as blueberries, strawberries, or raspberries)
- 1 tablespoon chia seeds
- 1 tablespoon unsweetened granola

Instructions:

1. The Greek yoghurt should be layered in half in a glass or bowl.

2. Add half of the mixed berries on top of the yoghurt.

3. Sprinkle half of the chia seeds and granola.

4. Repeat the layers with the remaining ingredients.

5. Enjoy!

Nutritional value per serving:

Calories: 250

Protein: 20g

Fat: 10g

Carbohydrates: 20g

Fibre: 7g

Veggie Sticks with Hummus

Preparation time: 10 minutes

Servings: 2

Ingredients:

- 2 medium-sized carrots
- 2 medium-sized cucumbers
- 1/2 cup hummus (store-bought or homemade)

Instructions:

1. Wash and peel the carrots and cucumbers.

2. Cut the carrots and cucumbers into sticks.

3. Serve with hummus as a dipping sauce.

Nutritional value per serving:

Calories: 120

Protein: 5g

Fat: 6g

Carbohydrates: 15g

Fibre: 6g

Almond Butter Energy Balls

Preparation time: 15 minutes

Servings: 12

Ingredients:

- 1 cup almond butter
- 1/2 cup rolled oats
- 1/4 cup honey or maple syrup
- 1/4 cup unsweetened shredded coconut
- 1/4 cup dark chocolate chips
- 1/4 cup chopped almonds

Instructions:

1. In a mixing bowl, combine almond butter, rolled oats, honey (or maple syrup), shredded coconut, dark chocolate chips, and chopped almonds.

2. Ensure all the ingredients are thoroughly mixed

3. Take small portions of the mixture and roll them into bite-sized balls using your hands.

4. Put the energy balls on a plate or baking sheet that has been parchment paper-lined.

5. Allow them to firm up in the refrigerator for a minimum of thirty minutes.

6. The energy balls can be consumed once they have chilled.

Nutritional value per serving (1 energy ball):

Calories: 150

Protein: 4g

Fat: 11g

Carbohydrates: 10g

Fibre: 3g

Kale Chips

Preparation time: 10 minutes

Cooking time: 15 minutes

Servings: 2

Ingredients:

- 1 bunch of kale
- 1 tablespoon olive oil
- 1/2 teaspoon sea salt
- 1/2 teaspoon paprika (optional)

Instructions:

1. Preheat the oven to 350°F (175°C).

2. Wash the kale leaves thoroughly and pat them dry.

3. The kale leaves should be stripped of their tough stems and torn into bite-sized pieces.

4. In a bowl, drizzle the kale leaves with olive oil and sprinkle with sea salt and paprika (if desired). Toss well to coat.

5. On a baking sheet covered with parchment paper, arrange the kale leaves in a single layer.

6. Bake for 12-15 minutes or until the kale leaves become crispy and slightly browned.

7. Prior to serving, take them out of the oven and let them cool down.

Nutritional value per serving:

Calories: 70

Protein: 4g

Fat: 4g

Carbohydrates: 8g

Fibre: 2g

Berry Protein Smoothie

Preparation time: 5 minutes

Servings: 1

Ingredients:

- one cup of almond milk or other non-dairy milk without sugar
- Half cup frozen mixed berries which includes strawberries, blueberries, and raspberries.
- 1/2 medium-sized banana
- 1 scoop of protein powder (plant-based or whey protein)
- 1 tablespoon chia seeds (optional)

- Ice cubes (optional)

Instructions:

1. In a blender, combine almond milk, frozen mixed berries, banana, protein powder, and chia seeds (if using).

2. Blend on high until smooth and creamy.

3. If desired, add a few ice cubes and blend again until well combined.

4. Pour into a glass and enjoy immediately.

Nutritional value per serving:

Calories: 250

Protein: 20g

Fat: 5g

Carbohydrates: 30g

Fibre: 8g

Berry Chia Pudding

Preparation time: 10 minutes

Servings: 2

Ingredients:

- 1 cup unsweetened almond milk

- 2 tablespoons chia seeds

- 1/2 teaspoon vanilla extract

- 1 cup mixed berries (strawberries, blueberries, raspberries)

- 1 tablespoon honey (optional)

Instructions:

1. In a bowl, combine almond milk, chia seeds, and vanilla extract. Stir well.

2. Let the mixture sit for 5 minutes, stirring occasionally to prevent clumps.

3. Divide the chia pudding into two serving glasses or jars.

4. Top with mixed berries and drizzle honey on top if desired.

5. Refrigerate for at least 2 hours or overnight to allow the chia seeds to expand and create a pudding-like consistency.

6. Serve chilled.

Nutritional value per serving:

Calories: 150

Carbohydrates: 18g

Protein: 5g

Fat: 7g

Fibre: 11g

Baked Apple with Cinnamon

Preparation time: 20 minutes

Servings: 1

Ingredients:

- 1 medium-sized apple
- 1/2 teaspoon cinnamon
- 1 teaspoon coconut oil
- 1 tablespoon chopped almonds

Instructions:

1. Preheat the oven to 350°F (180°C).

2. Cut the apple in half and remove the core.

3. Place the apple halves on a baking sheet.

4. Sprinkle cinnamon over the apple halves and drizzle with coconut oil.

5. Bake in the oven for 15 minutes or until the apple is soft.

6. Remove from the oven and sprinkle chopped almonds on top.

7. Serve warm.

Nutritional value per serving:

Calories: 170

Carbohydrates: 30g

Protein: 2g

Fat: 7g

Fibre: 6g

Chocolate Avocado Mousse

Preparation time: 15 minutes

Servings: 2

Ingredients:

- 1 ripe avocado
- 2 tablespoons unsweetened cocoa powder
- 2 tablespoons honey or maple syrup
- 1/2 teaspoon vanilla extract
- 1/4 cup unsweetened almond milk

Instructions:

1. In a blender or food processor, combine avocado, cocoa powder, honey or maple syrup, vanilla extract, and almond milk.

2. Blend until smooth and creamy.

3. Divide the mousse into two serving glasses or bowls.

4. Set and chill in the refrigerator for at least an hour.

5. Serve chilled.

Nutritional value per serving:

Calories: 180

Carbohydrates:12g

Protein: 3g

Fat: 11g

Fibre: 6g

Baked Peaches with Yogurt

Preparation time: 25 minutes

Servings: 2

Ingredients:

- 2 peaches, halved and pitted
- 1 tablespoon honey or maple syrup
- 1/2 teaspoon cinnamon
- 1/4 cup chopped walnuts
- 1/2 cup plain Greek yoghurt

Instructions:

1. Preheat the oven to 375°F (190°C).

2. Place the peach halves on a baking sheet, cut side up.

3. Drizzle honey or maple syrup over each peach half.

4. Sprinkle cinnamon and chopped walnuts on top.

5. Bake in the oven for 20 minutes or until the peaches are tender.

6. Take them out of the oven, and allow them cool a little.

7. Serve each peach half with a dollop of Greek yoghurt on top.

8. Enjoy warm.

Nutritional value per serving:

Calories: 180

Carbohydrates: 22g

Protein: 6g

Fat: 8g

Fibre: 3g

Coconut Flour Blueberry Muffins

Preparation time: 25 minutes

Servings: 6 muffins

Ingredients:

- 1/2 cup coconut flour
- 1/2 teaspoon baking powder
- 1/4 teaspoon salt
- 4 eggs
- 1/4 cup unsweetened almond milk
- 2 tablespoons coconut oil, melted
- 1/4 cup honey or maple syrup
- 1/2 teaspoon vanilla extract
- 1/2 cup blueberries

Instructions:

1. Set a muffin pan with paper liners and turn on the oven to 35 degree F(180 degree Celsius)

2. Coconut flour, baking powder, and salt should all be combined in a bowl.

3. In a separate bowl, beat the eggs, almond milk, coconut oil, honey or maple syrup, and vanilla extract.

4. Then, combine the dry ingredients thoroughly before adding the wet ingredients.

5. Gently fold in the blueberries.

6. Every muffin cup should receive an equal amount of batter.

7. Bake for eighteen to twenty minutes, or until a toothpick placed in the center comes out clean, in the preheated oven.

8. After letting the muffins cool for a short while in the pan, remove them and let them finish cooling on a wire rack.

Nutritional value per serving (1 muffin):

Calories: 160

Carbohydrates: 15g

Protein: 5g

Fat: 9g

Fibre: 4g

CHAPTER 6

Turmeric Ginger Tea

Ingredients:

- 1 teaspoon turmeric powder
- 1 teaspoon grated ginger
- 1 tablespoon lemon juice
- 1 teaspoon raw honey (optional)
- 2 cups hot water

Instructions:

1. Steep turmeric powder and grated ginger in hot water for 5 minutes.

2. Add lemon juice and honey. Stir well and enjoy.

Chia Seed Pudding

Ingredients:

- 2 tablespoons chia seeds
- 1 cup unsweetened almond milk
- 1/2 teaspoon vanilla extract

- 1 tablespoon chopped nuts (e.g., almonds, walnuts)
- Fresh berries for topping

Instructions:

1. Mix chia seeds, almond milk, and vanilla extract. Let it sit for 15 minutes, stirring occasionally.

2. Top with chopped nuts and fresh berries.

Hibiscus Iced Tea

Ingredients:

- 2 cups water
- 2 hibiscus tea bags
- 1 tablespoon honey (optional)
- Ice cubes

Instructions:

1. Bring water to a boil, then remove from heat. Ten minutes of hot water should be used to steep hibiscus tea bags.

2. Stir in honey if desired. Cool and serve over ice.

Coconut Water Smoothie

Ingredients:

- 1 cup coconut water

- 1/2 cup frozen pineapple chunks

- 1/2 cup frozen mango chunks

- 1/2 banana

- 1 tablespoon shredded coconut (unsweetened)

Instructions:

1. Blend all the ingredients until smooth. Add more coconut water if needed.

Green Smoothie

Ingredients:

- One cup of non-dairy milk of your choice, such as unsweetened almond milk
- 1 cup fresh spinach leaves
- 1/2 medium avocado
- 1/2 small banana
- 1 tablespoon chia seeds
- 1 tablespoon almond butter
- Optional: a few drops of liquid stevia or a natural sweetener of your choice (if desired)
- Ice cubes

Instructions:

2. In a blender, combine the almond milk, spinach leaves, avocado, banana, chia seeds, almond butter, and sweetener (if using).

3. Blend on high speed until all the ingredients are well combined and the smoothie has a creamy texture.

4. If the smoothie is too thick, add a little more almond milk until you reach your desired consistency.

5. Add a handful of ice cubes and blend again to chill the smoothie.

6. Pour into a glass and serve immediately as a refreshing and energizing drink.

CHAPTER 7

BONUS RECIPES FOR SPECIAL OCCASIONS AND HOLIDAYS

1. Sesame Tofu and Broccoli

Cooking time: 30 minutes

Servings: 4

Ingredients:

- One extra-firm block of tofu drained and pressed.
- One teaspoon of sesame oil
- One teaspoon of soy sauce
- One teaspoon of grated ginger
- one teaspoon of minced garlic
- Half a teaspoon of Black pepper
- One broccoli head cut into florets
- A quarter cup of finely chopped green onions

Instructions:

1. Adjust the temperature of the oven to 400 degrees F (200 degrees C).

2. Sesame oil, soy sauce, ginger, garlic, and black pepper should all be combined in a bowl.

3. Add the tofu, which has been cut into 1-inch cubes, to the marinade-containing bowl. Stir to coat.

4. On a baking sheet, layer the tofu and broccoli evenly.

5. Bake the broccoli and tofu for 20 to 25 minutes, or until they are both cooked through.

6. Serve after adding green onions.

Nutritional value:

Calories: 290

Fat: 17 grams

Protein: 18 grams

Carbohydrates: 15 grams

2. Farro Mushroom Risotto

Cooking time: 30 minutes

Servings: 4

Ingredients:

- One cup of Farro
- Half a cup of white wine
- Four cups of chicken or vegetable broth
- A quarter cup of olive oil
- One chopped onion
- Two minced garlic cloves
- one pound of sliced mushrooms
- a half-cup of chopped Parmesan cheese.
- salt and pepper for seasoning

Instructions:

1. Allow the broth to boil together in a saucepan.

2. In a big skillet over medium flame, liquefy the olive oil.

3. It ought to be soft five minutes after the onion is added.

4. Put the garlic and fry for another minute.

5. The mushrooms should be added to the skillet and cooked for about 5 minutes, or until soft.

6. As soon as you add the farro, stir it to evenly distribute the oil. It takes about 2 minutes to absorb the wine after adding it to the pan.

7. The farro will absorb the hot broth after receiving 1 cup of it.

8. For about 20 minutes, until the farro is fully cooked and the risotto is creamy, add the broth a cup at a time while continuously stirring.

9. Add the Parmesan cheese and taste-test adding salt and pepper.

10. Serve instantly.

Nutritional value:

Calories: 380

Fat: 14 grams

Protein: 12 grams

Carbohydrates: 50 grams

3. Vegan Palak Tofu

Cooking time: 30 minutes

Servings: 4

Ingredients:

- One extra-firm block of tofu drained and pressed.

- One teaspoon of olive oil

- one sliced onion

- Two cloves of crushed garlic

- One teaspoon of cumin powder

- Half a teaspoon of turmeric

- A quarter teaspoon of cayenne pepper

- One can of drained diced tomatoes

- One package of thawed and drained frozen spinach

- Salt and pepper for seasoning

Instructions:

1. Adjust the temperature of the oven to 175 degrees Celsius) at 350 degrees Fahrenheit.

2. In a big skillet over medium flame, liquefy the olive oil.

3. It ought to be soft five minutes after the onion is added. Put the garlic and fry for another minute.

4. Cook for another minute after adding the cumin, turmeric, and cayenne.

5. Add the tofu, spinach, and tomatoes after that. Ten minutes should pass after bringing it to a simmer so that the sauce has had time to thicken.

6. When seasoning, season to taste with pepper and salt.

7. Bake the mixture in a baking dish for 20 minutes, or until the tofu is thoroughly heated.

Nutritional value:

Calories: 350

Fat: 16 grams

Protein: 2

4. Buddha Bowl

Cooking time: 30 minutes

Servings: 1

Ingredients:

- One cooked cup of brown rice
- Half a cup of cooked quinoa

- Half a cup of roasted Vegetables like broccoli, carrots, and sweet potatoes
- A quarter cup of black beans
- A quarter cup of corn
- A quarter cup of salsa
- A quarter cup of avocado
- A quarter cup of chopped cilantro
- Salt and pepper for seasoning

Instructions:

1. Combine the black beans, corn, salsa, avocado, cilantro, quinoa, roasted vegetables, and brown rice in a sizable bowl.

2. When seasoning, season to taste with pepper and salt

3. Serve instantly.

Nutritional value:

Calories: 500

Fat: 15 grams

Protein: 20 grams

Carbohydrates: 75 grams

5. Creamy Vegan Korma

Cooking time: 30 minutes

Servings: 4

Ingredients:

- One teaspoon of olive oil

- One sliced onion

- Two cloves of finely chopped garlic

- one teaspoon of powdered turmeric

- half a teaspoon of cumin powder

- Cayenne pepper, 1/4 teaspoon

- One can of diced tomatoes without the drain

- One can of Coconut milk

- 10 ounces of frozen cauliflower florets, thawed and drained, in one package

- Salt and pepper for seasoning

Instructions:

1. In a big skillet over medium flame, liquefy the olive oil.

2. The onion should be soft after adding it and cooking for about 5 minutes. Put the garlic and fry for another minute.

3. Cook for another minute after adding the cayenne, cumin, and turmeric to the skillet.

4. Add salt and pepper to taste along with the tomatoes, coconut milk, and cauliflower.

5. The cauliflower should be cooked for 20 minutes, or until it is tender, at a simmer.

6. Serve the food hot.

Nutritional value:

Calories: 400

Fat: 25 grams

Protein: 10 grams

Carbohydrates: 35 grams

I Hope You Enjoy These Recipes!

CONCLUSION

Embracing the PCOS Diet for a Healthier You

Although Polycystic Ovary Syndrome (PCOS) can be a difficult condition to manage, it is possible to live a healthier and happier life by making the appropriate dietary and lifestyle changes. You can control your symptoms and enhance your general health and well-being by adhering to the PCOS diet.

Making healthy decisions that support your body's needs is the foundation of the PCOS diet. Consuming a balanced diet that is high in whole foods like fruits, vegetables, lean proteins, and healthy fats is necessary to achieve this. Additionally, it entails staying away from processed foods, sweetened beverages, and bad fats that can exacerbate insulin resistance and inflammation.

A healthy diet and regular exercise are both essential for managing PCOS. Exercise can improve insulin sensitivity, lower stress levels, and help you maintain a healthy weight. Most days of the week, try to get in at least 30 minutes of moderate-intensity exercise. Include activities you enjoy, like walking, swimming, or yoga.

The PCOS diet also emphasizes getting enough sleep and controlling stress. Prioritizing self-care activities like meditation, deep breathing exercises, or soothing hobbies is crucial because lack of sleep and ongoing stress can disrupt hormone levels and worsen PCOS symptoms.

You can take charge of your health and enhance your quality of life by adopting the PCOS diet and changing your way of life. Remember to seek personalized advice on managing PCOS through dietary and lifestyle changes from a healthcare professional or registered dietitian.

Don't let PCOS prevent you from leading the best life possible. Take the first step toward a healthier you by adopting the PCOS diet!